Age, not a barrier:

The Longevity Therapy Manual
By

Josh S. Morton

Age, not a barrier

Table of content

Age, not a barrier

Book Review

Aging has for some time been seen as a natural occurrence. We believe that illness, weakness, and progressive decline are inevitable parts of life, but this is not so because science considers aging to be a treatable condition. By addressing the root causes, we can not only improve our health and live longer but also prevent and reverse diseases associated with aging, including depression, heart disease, cancer, diabetes, and Dementia. In **"Age, not a Barrier", Dr. Josh S. Morton** challenges us to review our biology, health, and aging. To uncover the secrets of longevity, he explores the biological features of aging, their causes, and consequences, then shows us how to overcome them with diets, lifestyle simplicity, and emerging longevity strategies. You'll learn how to optimize your body's key longevity switches; reduce inflammation and support your immune system health. Exercise, sleep, mental health, fitness, and enriching your social relationships are explored in different ways to achieve optimal aging outcomes. You'll also get a look into **Dr. Josh S. Morton's** explanations on how to age without stress. With dozens of science-backed strategies and tips, **"Age, not a Barrier"** is a profound practical guide to creating a path to a healthy, and general well-being.

Age, not a barrier

The main goal of this book is to ensure that the aging process proceeds healthily through a complete presentation of everything necessary.
Click on the **buy** button now to get the opportunity to read the unequalled depth on Longevity in good health and optimum fitness.

Introduction

Longevity is the result of living a long life. We all hope to live long so we can spend years of quality time with our loved ones and have time to explore the world. However, reaching old age does not necessarily mean being healthy and happy. If you need to live long, you must plan to avoid getting sick. The number of people over 65 is growing faster than any other age group due to longer life expectancies and lower birth rates, but people are spending more years in poor health, therefore we will examine not only life expectancy but also healthy life expectancy. What you do today can change your health and future age. Ideally, you should start early, but even if you start late, it's never too late to reap the benefits. This book highlights key areas you can focus on to improve your health. Exercise, diet, sleep, mental health, and social environment remain the base to improving our health. Although there is hardly a clear pattern for achieving longevity, this book attempts to harmonize the important aspects that

Age, not a barrier

will ensure that you can achieve your goals of not only living a long life but also remaining fitness to stay strong and healthy.

Key idea 1

What Exercise Does

Constant exercise is known to raise energy levels and improve mood. It may also be associated with many other powerful health benefits, including reduced risk of chronic diseases. Exercise is any movement that works your muscles and causes your body to burn calories. There are many different types of physical activities such as swimming, running, jogging, walking, and dancing, to name a few. Being active has been proven to have many health benefits, both physically and mentally, and ultimately leads to a longer life. Exercising plays a role in improving one's excitement and reducing the likelihood for depression, anxiety, and stress, this is done by ensuring some changes to parts of the brain responsible for the control of stress and anxiety. It can also increase the brain's

Age, not a barrier

sensitivity to serotonin and noradrenaline, hormones that relieve feelings of depression. Additionally, exercise can increase the production of endorphins, which are known to produce positive feelings and help reduce pain perception. Strength training and weight lifting are important for everyone, including the elderly and frail. It can improve your mobility and physical performance and help prevent falls and other health problems in old age, but if you don't feel like you have the time or funds to continue this form of exercise, a simple exercise plan may be all you need. Exercising without paying attention to intensity can improve your mood and blood flow. Consider this as a starting point.
You may not need to meet the global minimum recommendations of 30 minutes of exercise a day, five times a week, to extend your lifespan.
One study found that 15 minutes of moderate-intensity exercise per day increased the lifespan of participants by three years. This finding also applies to people with health problems, such as cardiovascular disease, and overweight people who don't lose weight while being active in the study. Brisk walking was

Age, not a barrier

one of the "moderate-intensity" exercises mentioned in the study. It may take a conscious effort to incorporate it into your daily life, but 15 minutes of exercise can help you live an extra three years, which seems like a pretty good bargain for longevity. It's no surprise that physical activity can maintain health and extend lifespan. Just 15 minutes of exercise per day can add up to three years to your life. Additionally, each additional 15 minutes of daily physical activity reduces your risk of premature death by 4%. A recent study found that people who exercised had a 22% lower risk of premature death, even if they did less than the recommended 150 minutes per week. Those who met the 150-minute recommendation had a 28% lower risk of premature death. Furthermore, this figure was 35% for those who exercised beyond these guidelines.

Key idea 2

Importance of fitness

Physical activity is the movement of the body produced by skeletal muscles that results in energy expenditure. Energy expenditure can be measured in kilocalories. Physical activity in daily life can be grouped into occupational, sports, conditioning, domestic, or other activities.
Exercise is a part of physical activity that is planned, organized, and performed repeatedly, with the ultimate or intermediate goal of increasing or maintaining physical fitness.

Age, not a barrier

Being physically fit encompasses some attributes which are related to preventing diseases and ensuring a wholesome wellbeing. Therefore, it is common and appropriate to measure components of physical fitness before preventive and rehabilitation programs. Physical fitness can be achieved through regular physical activity, healthy eating, and exercise. Physical fitness has been shown to have a significant positive correlation with physical activity and effective nutrition, which in turn extends lifespan.

What fitness does

Muscle strength

It is the "power" needed to lift or carry heavy objects. Without muscle strength, the body becomes weak and unable to meet the demands placed on it. The way to increase muscle strength is to use heavy weights to train. The more heavy the weight is, the lesser reps should be done.

Muscular endurance

Endurance is the ability of muscles to contract for long periods. Rather than just lifting or carrying something for a few seconds, your muscles are stressed for several minutes. A way to increase muscle strength is to train with light weights in the range of 20-25 repetitions. Working with lighter weights trains the muscle fibers needed for muscular endurance, and increasing your rep range increases your training time.

Cardiovascular endurance

Cardiovascular endurance is the body's ability to withstand exercise such as running, jogging, swimming, cycling, and any exercise that puts strain on the cardiovascular system (lungs, heart, and blood vessels). The heart and lungs work together to supply your body with the oxygen your muscles need to do their work. The Cooper Run (running as far as you can in 12 minutes) is a commonly used test to assess cardiovascular endurance. However, many trainers also use the step test (stepping on a platform for 5 minutes). Both are accurate measurements of a subject's endurance.

Flexibility

Flexibility is one of the most important elements of physical fitness, but it is often overlooked. Without flexibility, your muscles and joints will become stiff and your movement will be restricted. Flexibility training ensures that you can perform a full range of motion in your body without feeling pain or stiffness. To test your flexibility, try leaning forward and touching your toes. People with high flexibility can usually touch their toes, while people with low flexibility

cannot. The sit-and-reach test (sitting on the floor with a stretched leg and reaching for your toes) is also a good way to assess flexibility. The more flexible you are, the more you can touch your toes and beyond.

Composition of body fat

The amount of fats within the body is known as Body fat composition. For example, a person who weighs 100 pounds and has 25% body fat has 75 pounds of lean body mass. Men should have less than 17% body fat. Women must have less than 24% body fat. The average male body fat percentage

relative to a female is usually around 18-24%, while the average female body fat percentage is 25-31%.

Key idea 3

Wholesome Dieting

Wholesome dieting as other factors is integral and always important to having a longspan of life, let's look at everything diet-related. A major problem facing Western world today is poor eating habit which originates from the components of foods eaten. Most foods contain high levels of sugar and other refined nutritional additives which when eaten in large quantities overtime results in poor health. There is currently a lot of concern about the link

Age, not a barrier

between calorie intake and longevity. Animal studies show that reducing normal calorie intake by 10 to 50 percent can increase maximum lifespan. Studies of human populations known for their longevity have also observed a link between low-calorie intake with extended lifespan and lower risk of disease. Additionally, calorie restriction helps reduce excess weight and belly fat, two factors linked to a shorter lifespan. That said, long-term calorie restriction is often unsustainable and can lead to negative side effects, such as increased hunger, low body temperature, and decreased libido; This is the most flexible option but requires you to track everything you eat and resist the urge to cheat. Dietary restriction involves cutting out specific foods but only works if it results in a time-restricted calorie deficit, such as intermittent fasting; which can be counterproductive if you eat too much after the fast or don't get enough protein.

Age, not a barrier

Let's turn the tables for a minute and focus on what you should be eating.
Eating a variety of plant foods, such as fruits, vegetables, nuts, seeds, whole
grains, and beans, can reduce disease risk and increase longevity. Many studies
link plant-rich diets to a reduced risk of premature death as well as a reduced
risk of cancer, metabolic syndrome, heart disease, depression, and brain
damage. These effects are due to plant foods containing safe nutrients and
antioxidants, including polyphenols, carotenoids, folate, and vitamin C. Nuts are
also essential and can be described as nutritional powerhouse since they are rich
in protein, fiber, antioxidants, and other beneficial plant compounds; they are
also an excellent reservoir of many other minerals, and vitamins the likes of
copper, potassium,folate, and vitamins B6 and E. Some studies show that nuts
have beneficial effects on heart disease, high blood pressure, inflammation,
diabetes, metabolic syndrome, belly fat, and even some forms of cancer.
Fats, they are an important part of your diet, but some are healthier than others.
Choosing healthy fats from plant sources more often than less healthy fats from

Age, not a barrier

animal products can help reduce your risk of heart attack, stroke, and other serious health problems. Foods high in bad (saturated) fats are animal products such as butter, cheese, whole milk, ice cream, and fatty meats; Some vegetable oils such as coconut oil, palm oil, and palm kernel oil also contain saturated fats. Diets high in saturated fat increase cholesterol buildup in the arteries (blood vessels). Cholesterol is a soft, wax-like substance that can clog or block arteries. A good fats healthy diet is essential in ensuring high levels of fitness, which ultimately leads to longevity.

Key idea 4

Good sleep habit

Sleep is important for regulating cellular function and helping your body recover. A recent study reports that longevity may be related to regular sleep habits, such as going to bed and waking up at the same time every day. Sleep duration also appears to be a factor, as too little or too much sleep is harmful. For example, sleeping fewer hours per night is associated with a 12% higher risk of premature death, while sleeping too long each night can also reduce your life expectancy by up to 38%. Too little sleep promotes inflammation and increases your risk of diabetes, heart disease, and obesity. All this is associated with a shortened lifespan. Anxiety and stress can also be caused by lack of sleep, which can lead to a significant reduction in your lifespan. For example, women with stress or anxiety are twice as likely to die from heart disease, stroke, or lung cancer. Similarly, the risk of early death in anxious or stressed men is three times higher than in more relaxed men. If you feel stressed, sleep and optimism can be important parts of the solution. Studies show that pessimistic people are 42% more likely to die prematurely than more optimistic people. However, sleep and a positive outlook on life can reduce stress and potentially prolong your life. It's important to note that stress damages longevity in two ways. The first is due to the direct impact of stress on your body in the long term, stress triggers the release of a hormone called cortisol that helps you respond to threats by increasing your heart rate and breathing rate, long-term elevations can be harmful and can result in depression, high blood pressure, anxiety, and other heart diseases. Secondly, there is also evidence that prolonged stress can "age" cells at the molecular level. On the other hand, sleeping too much may be linked to depression, lack of physical activity, and undiagnosed health conditions, all of which can negatively affect your longevity. This therefore requires creating a workable balance to provide for necessary required sleep which should be between 6 and 9hrs at night.

Key idea 5

Sound mental health

Emotional, psychological, and social well-being are all components of our mental health. Our mental health influences most of our actions . It also helps shape how we manage stress, interact with others, and make healthy choices. Mental health is important at every stage of life, from childhood to adolescence to adulthood. Both mental and physical health are integral components of our overall health or well being. For example, depression increases the risk of many types of physical health problems, especially chronic diseases such as diabetes, heart disease, and stroke. Likewise, the presence of chronic diseases may increase the risk of mental illness, implying that mental health may play an important role in a person's life and therefore should be addressed. In the United States, more than one in five adults live with mental illness. More than one in five young people (ages 13-18), now or at some point in their lives, suffer from a seriously debilitating mental illness. About 1 in 25 people in the United States adults are living with serious mental illness, such as schizophrenia, bipolar disorder, or major depression. There is no single cause of mental illness. Several factors may contribute to the risk of mental illness, such as adverse childhood experiences such as trauma or a history of violence (e.g., child abuse, sexual assault, witnessing violence, etc. Biological factors or chemical imbalances in the brain can also cause mental health imbalances, with alcohol or drug use being other causes of poor mental health.

How to improve your mental health

Feeling happy can significantly increase your lifespan. A study showed the happiest people saw a decrease in premature death over a five-year study period. A study of 180 Catholic nuns analyzed their reported happiness levels when they first entered the convent and then compared those levels to their life expectancy. People who feel happiest at age 22 are more likely to still be alive six decades later.

Age, not a barrier

Conscientiousness refers to a person's ability to be disciplined, organized, efficient, and goal-oriented. According to data from a study that followed 1,500 boys and girls into old age, children who were considered persistent, organized, and disciplined lived 11 percent longer than their less conscientious counterparts. Conscientious people may also have lower blood pressure and fewer mental problems, as well as a lower risk of diabetes and heart or joint problems. This may partly be because conscientious individuals are less likely to take dangerous risks or react negatively to stress - and are more likely to lead successful lives in their careers or take charge of their health. Consciousness can be developed at any stage of life through small steps like cleaning your desk, following a work schedule, or being on time.

Anger can be a difficult emotion to express, especially if you feel your outrage is justified. Perhaps the better question to ask yourself is: Is it worth the Cortisol? Levels of this stress hormone increase when you are stressed or angry, causing negative effects on your heart, metabolism, and immune system. Very high cortisol amount is associated to increased mortality in general.

Take life a step at a time, radical lifestyle changes can be inspiring but can also be scary – and therefore short-lived – for the average person. Next time you decide to eat healthier or exercise more, try setting a lower goal. Try choosing just one small change at a time, such as waking up 10 minutes earlier in the morning to prepare a healthy lunch for work, rather than attempting to make a big change in your life all at once. As the exercise tips above show, even short bursts of daily activity can have big benefits for your longevity. Small changes can go unnoticed, delivering big benefits over time without putting a strain on your busy world. Consistency is more important than a short-term gesture. Additionally, checking in on what's already working in your daily routine can

Age, not a barrier

help you feel energized and motivated to push a little more in a healthy direction.

Key idea 6

Nurture your social circle

Researchers report that maintaining a healthy social network can help you live up to 50% longer. Having just 3 social ties can significantly reduce the risk of premature death. There is a connection between a healthy social network to right changes in heart, brain, hormonal, and immune function, which reduce the vulnerability to chronic diseases. A strong social network may also help you react less negatively to stress, perhaps further explaining the positive impact on longevity. Socializing can be a good longevity booster, mainly by helping you manage stress and boost your immune system. Good relationships keep you

Age, not a barrier

strong, while bad relationships can make you think negatively and put you at risk for depression and even heart failure. Associating with people or maintaining a healthy social circle could be an issue if you're depressed, experienced the demise of a loved one, or stay far from family and and loved ones. There are many ways to reconnect or meet new people even when you're in a new city, including volunteering and connecting with others with similar interests through networks like business groups and book clubs. Finally, one study reports that supporting others may be more beneficial than receiving that support. In addition to accepting care from friends and family, make sure you reciprocate.

Final summary

Longevity may seem out of your control, but many healthy habits can lead you to a ripe old age with a stronger bodily build. As we have seen in this text, longevity can be improved by several factors: physical activities and regular exercise promote healthy blood circulation and brain function, but even small amounts of exercise can also help. Eating plenty of plant foods, proteins, healthy fats, and calorie discipline helps reduce the risk of various common diseases. Developing sleep habits that include 6 to 9 hours of sleep each night will increase cognitive

Age, not a barrier

awareness. Finding ways to reduce your anxiety and stress levels will help reduce your risk of depression or injury. Maintaining close relationships can help reduce stress levels and improve immunity.
Together, these habits can improve your health and put you on the path toward longevity.